The Nations Health

The Nations Health

*The Necessary Revolution Towards
A Healthy Nation*

Ernest Roberts

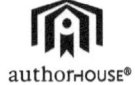

authorHOUSE®

AuthorHouse™
1663 Liberty Drive
Bloomington, IN 47403
www.authorhouse.com
Phone: 1-800-839-8640

First published by AuthorHouse   07/25/2011

ISBN: 978-1-4567-8618-2 (sc)
ISBN: 978-1-4567-8619-9 (ebk)

Printed in the United States of America

*Any people depicted in stock imagery provided by Thinkstock are models,
and such images are being used for illustrative purposes only.
Certain stock imagery © Thinkstock.*

This book is printed on acid-free paper.

*Because of the dynamic nature of the Internet, any web addresses or
links contained in this book may have changed since publication and
may no longer be valid. The views expressed in this work are solely those
of the author and do not necessarily reflect the views of the publisher,
and the publisher hereby disclaims any responsibility for them.*

For Andrew Wakefield

Acknowledgments

I have been supported and informed by many who have in their writings shown knowledge, experience and common sense.

I am especially indebted to Dr. Paul Goddard's insights into the fragility of the Welfare State, or "welfare myth" as he mentions.

John Humphry's "The Great Food Gamble" and the works of Felicity Lawrence reveal the dangers of transforming traditional, natural food provision into an industry where the laws of mass production and 'profit at all costs' are borrowed from manufacturing.

Principles of cooking and diet based on the observation of and the respect for nature are given by George Ohsawa's books on macrobiotics which describe traditional family methods of food preparation and cooking uncontaminated by commercial vested interests or by the influence of scientific theories and research far distanced from nature. Macrobiotics relates diet and cooking to universal principles of energy and the relationship between food and health based on the observation of nature.

Thanks to Gordon Ellis, Psychotherapist, for his advice and information on Mental Health Treatment. Thanks to my friend Professor John D. Pearson for his helpful advice on the first draft and proof reading. Also to Elizabeth Bogden, Homoeopathic Practitioner who previously worked for many years in the Pharmaceutical Industry, who has given me the references on medical drugs and their regulation that I have researched for this work. Thanks to Jerome Whitney for the advice and recipes on diets and cleansing regimes.

1

Introduction

Health means whole, good health requires a whole view, it involves choices about all aspects of living including something as simple as the quality and quantity of food and drink we use.

Social Cost has to be accounted for in addition to the market price of goods. Cheap goods often come with the creation of additional costs which are borne by society as a whole and are paid for in higher national and local taxes.

Fear The Plague told me on its way to London, "I go to kill a thousand people. When he returned I chastised him "two thousand died not one"

"Yes" he responded, "but It was fear that killed the rest"

Fear is a great causation of illness and of wrong approaches to its treatment. In 2009 pharmaceutical companies banked £4.8 bn. When the NHS needlessly stockpiled swine flu vaccine. This decision was fed by fear rather than good judgement. Alleged bribery of scientific advisers was also implicated here.(1)

Fear inspires the belief that agents outside of your own chosen life style give you illness, for example germs, viruses and bacteria. Truly such entities exist but their ability to harm depends entirely on each person's individual susceptibility and come into the body only when there are suitable conditions to attract and feed them, the "terrain".

Fear also allows you to overuse treatments of all kinds. Medicines which influence hormones require especial care. Many so called safe medicines have been withdrawn for safety fears.

Unnecessary vaccinations and surgery can also cause ill health.

<u>Self Reliance</u>

Resilience to disease and the power of your immunity depends to a great extent on the quality of your daily thought patterns and the quality of your emotions. Negative, worrying, anxious and fearful thoughts weaken your immunity, positive thoughts achieve the reverse.

Thoughts and emotions control secretions from the main ductless glands. The balance of these chemical messengers regulates every organ and system in your body. These emotional and mental causes of illness are more important than many physical ones.

D. A. Kessler (2) details research which shows how chemical secretions in our brains make us desire harmful foods and to over eat them, this is good exoteric science. However it is our thoughts, feelings, attitudes and choices which determine these very chemical secretions and we can control these, this is esoteric science. Right thought is an ability to determine action and dominate the situation. Animals, being closer to nature often choose a healthy regime, surplus food is buried or stored in other ways, so that excess is avoided. Kessler seems to be saying that a large proportion of people are less evolved than animals, they are slaves to their chemical secretions rather than master of them. Which of us are members of the 'Choosing People' and are in balance with our material world rather than subject to it?

It is clear that each individual must take responsibility for their own state of health and also how society nurtures health care. We cannot rely on others to do it for us. Vested interests have resources to influence the press, the government and to direct attention away from unpopular or uncomfortable choices and policies. Medical research is financed by drug companies to a large extent, conventional medicines are researched and sold to medics by companies which aim to optimise profits, in many cases to the detriment of patients.

"Rachel's Environment and Health Weekly" is a journal which details the intense pressure that drug company

sales staff put upon doctors and the large amount of money spent on the promotion of drugs:

Civilization. Certain tenets have been a part of the ethos of Western societies for several centuries. Indeed, origins of these principles can be traced to ancient civilizations in each of the continents of the world. These ideas include the rule of law and the necessity to have strong rulers who consider the welfare of the whole rather than merely their own self enhancement. Government had to be respected and trusted. We find expression of them in social and political philosophical texts like the Tau Te Ching, a book from ancient China. States do not need any particular form of government in preference to another, whether it is democracy, oligarchy or dictatorship. The state requires a stable authority to establish order, justice and peace so that people can work, live and flourish. If a country has a dictatorship there may be a good reason for this. The issue is whether the rule in beneficial or deleterious. Religion and spiritual teaching has always been a part of society and has provided guidance which furthered these ideas and the principle of service. In the nineteenth century the middle classes in England gave 10% of their income to charity.

In recent times organized religion has begun to fail in this beneficial influence. Excesses, hypocrisy, irrational beliefs and dogma characteristic of organized religion have allowed its authority to become weakened and have alienated peoples. The appeal of Humanist and rationalist critiques of religion have added to this decline. This has been compounded by the influence of the American lead culture of excess and violence. All this has led to an extensive rejection of religious authority leaving a vacuum in spiritual guidance and restraint on selfishness from our governments. When society is without moral codes behaviour tends towards being violent, uncontrolled and destructive. True spiritual teaching encourages self reliance and responsibility.

"Self reliance and meditation are better than prayer and petition."

Recent studies show conclusively that Spirituality is the key to children's happiness. (3)

2

The Origins of the Welfare State and the National Health Service

These were born from an altruistic endeavour to help those less privileged. The working classes had been exploited and degraded by a process of destroying self sufficient families and communities which began with the land enclosure movement and continued apace with the industrial revolution.

*The Capitalist Dilemma. It was John Maynard Keynes who paved the way for the Welfare State. After the trade cycles of the nineteenth century and the Great Depression of the 1930's Keynes showed how to manage a capitalist economy without excesses of poverty and uncertainty. His analysis of the economy showed the necessity for the state to either employ for wages or to pay financial benefits to the unemployed. **This was a revolution, it produced many positive effects but negatively it lead to the idea of the welfare state and the expectation among people that they need not be independent and self reliant, as the government would provide for them in all areas including income, education and healthcare.***

"The more subsidies you have the less self-reliant people will become" Tao Te Ching

Inevitably the same lack of responsibility by individuals affects all segments of society as we saw in 2007 in the case of bankers and financiers

The costs of bad living and eating—who should pay?

Overweight and obesity lead to illness. Diabetes is often mentioned but many other conditions, less or more serious can arise including kidney stones, high blood pressure, joint and back pains like lumbago and arthritis. Diet related disease is estimated to cost £6bn. A year (Guardian 13.11.10) Dementia has also been implicated by a team of British and French researchers who found that a better diet would reduce obesity and ultimately dementia. Guardian 6/8/2010. **In the light of the expectation that medical and social services are responsible for correcting and treating all ailments pressure is put on the public purse to finance this.** *Usual medical treatment is doomed to fail because cure vitally depends upon each patient making quite serious efforts to correct and reverse the progress of disease originating as it does to a great extent in bad life style, eating habits and diet.*

Additionally there is a rapid escalation of the cost of the National Health Service. In 1948 the NHS budget was £170 million, with no provision for any increase, assuming the population would become more healthy. The NHS now costs £100 billion per year. (4 P.66).(It is worth noting here that homoepathic medicines cost very little). This process has been progressing over the years putting pressure on its continued existence. Unless a completely new approach is adopted the principle of health care being provided to all will end in quite turbulent political and social change. It is clearly unfair that the whole population should pay for the consequences of individual's irresponsible choices of life style, diet etc.

Costs must be related to causes which means a complete rethink of both how medical care is financed and how disease is treated

Inequality of Income It is futile and misguided to try to solve the problem of inequality in the distribution of income by any other means than to address the problem directly. Medical practitioners and a health service should not be expected to operate so as to redistribute income.

The Illusion of Better Health Politicians and doctors frequently claim that the N.H.S. has produced good results, for example that people are living longer. What is not taken into account is the quality of life, a lack of independence and a reliance on medication which on balance produces a less healthy life condition.

"Modern medicine itself causes illness, over 6% of UK hospital admissions are directly caused by side-effects of prescribed drugs." (6)

3

The regulation, provision, and safety of medical drugs

Drugs are provided by a private, profit-motivated oligopoly over which there is no real control or regulation. Marcia Angell found that the pharmaceutical industry is the most profitable in the world. (7)

There is an economic law which states that the consumption of anything will continue until its value to the user is equal to its cost. (marginal utility equals marginal cost) When the cost is zero consumption will continue indefinitely. Free health care leaves no incentive to use alternative health treatments which were used for generations to prevent illness becoming too serious. Similarly people have no real need to pursue a life style which prevents illness when its treatment can be left to the free medical service. For these reasons the NHS faces an impossible task; in the society of today demand will always exceed supply, there is no need for this to be so.

One manifestation of this impasse are the frequent administrative change in the NHS, like the introduction of Primary Care Trusts (PCT's) which were set up to save money, these have now been abolished. The problems revealed by the way PCT's worked remain. Prescribing generic drugs is encouraged despite the fact that GP's prefer to prescribe branded drugs because they have tighter quality control, no doubt because of the fear of expensive law suits, they are much more expensive than generic drugs. Strategic Health Authorities have also been abolished leaving GP's to decide on treatments and allocate funds. **These new changes offer no hope of solving the fundamental problems of the NHS until individual patients are given responsibility for their own health and the real causes of illness addressed with the necessary reforms.**

<u>The National Institute of Clinical Excellence. (N.I.C.E.)</u>
The work of NICE has been surrounded by controversy since its inception in 1997. Its work is to review new drugs, their clinical efficacy and cost. NICE clinicians found themselves unable to tell which new products were most effective, leading to local variations in commissioning practices. At the heart of the majority of criticisms of NICE was the requirement that its decisions reflect the cost effectiveness of treatments which means that its clinical recommendations are inextricably tied up with political decisions about value for money.

It is stipulated that in all drug trials comities of independent experts should scrutinize data and warn, if necessary, that it was unsafe to carry on. Nottingham University researchers found that fewer than 2% of the 739 international drug trials published between 1996 and 2000 had comities and of these unscrutinized trials six had to be stopped early because of toxic effects on the child patients. (Guardian 2 May 2008) We all know that deaths have occurred during drug trials.

<u>Medicines and Healthcare Products Regulatory Authority M.H.P.R.A.</u> This is an executive agency of the Department of Health set up to ensure that medicines and medical devices work and are acceptably safe. They say that "no product is risk free, we try to ensure that the benefits to patients and the public justify the risks.

(Doubts have also been cast on the effectiveness of regulation of the food industry. See reference (8) pp. 293/4/5)

4

A record of prescribed drugs which were withdrawn

Often prescribed drugs, passed as safe by N.I.C.E. are later withdrawn. Hardly a month passes without a drug prescribed by doctors throughout the UK being withdrawn. Acomplia, a slimming drug aimed at treating obesity which "doubled the risk of psychiatric disorders" was withdrawn. The Guardian 24 October 2008. This is especially unacceptable because a similar slimming drug, Rimonaband also approved by N.I.C.E. was found to have effects like depression anxiety and suicidal tendencies and was withdrawn earlier the same year. Without treating the causes of obesity such drug treatment is bound to fail. Other withdrawn drugs were: Quitiapin, Viox, Arcoxia and Dextra. As you would expect the situation in America is similar. The American Food and Drug Agency in 1998 gives 59 drug products that have been removed from the market for reasons of safety and effectiveness between 1973 and 1983.(Federal Register October 8 1998 Vol. 63 No. 195).

"As big business holds the purse strings, there are far fewer grants available to examine the safety of new products than there are to approve them." (4)

Another report states that 51% of approved drugs have serious harmful effects not detected prior to approval and revealed that antipsychotic drugs kill 1,800 dementia sufferers every year at a cost of £55m. *Guardian* 13 November 2009.

5

The Causes of Disease

Acute illnesses are those that come, reach a peak and then go which is a sign of a healthy body responding in the best way to passing challenges of weather, environment or circumstances. Continual long term illness (chronic disease) is a process taking time to come to fruition and is largely the responsibility of each individual and the result of the choices we make or fail to make. Acute illnesses may be converted into deep chronic illness by wrong treatment.

SOCIAL CAUSES There are social factors underlying individual choices which come under the influence of intelligent government and social institutions:

"Only through implementing policies that help to reduce inequalities within our society and build resilience of individuals and communities will we engender the social, economic and health benefits that are the hallmarks of a healthy society" (5)

Simon Kuznets, the economist who helped to develop the concept of GDP believed that

"The Welfare of a nation can scarcely be inferred from a measure of the national income." (4)

Inequality of income. The large discrepancy in income and wealth across society is a dominant influence on the whole spectrum of social issues and choices of life style. Gross inequalities of income between groups and occupations feeds anti-social behaviour in many ways, influencing all aspects of self reliance and encouraging alienation within society. It feeds illness on the deepest level of spiritual ill health. The divergence is far more than can be explained by markets and social forces or just rewards for hard endeavour, skills and talent. Poverty will never be modified to a healthy proportion until the problem of excess wealth and income is tackled. In a detailed study of inequality the following nine areas were found to be affected: level of trust, mental illness, life expectancy, obesity, educational achievement, teenage births, homicides, imprisonment rates and social mobility. (9) A Zen aphorism says whatever has a front has a back, the bigger the front the bigger the back. poverty is the back of wealth.

Religion, Wealth and Poverty Christianity pays lip service to equality. The testaments preach sermons urging us not to hoard goods and wealth, the rich man is advised to sell his goods and give the money to the poor. Humility, modesty and equality are ideas which permeate Christianity. Despite this Christian countries value and tolerate gross inequality of all material goods and wealth.

Culture. The culture and background in which our individual choices are made, is relevant to one major influence on our health namely the degree to which we indulge in alcohol, tobacco and other harmful, non food substances in which I include recreational and prescribed drugs. (10) It is important which media we read or watch which affects the likely impact of advertising and commercial dominance on our ideas about food, diet, nutrition and life style.

Education Over emphasis on mental development during schooling whilst neglecting emotional needs often leads to illness at some stage including mental illness.

A detailed assessment of the importance of social factors can be found in an E.U. Commission report on a new way of approaching social progress (10). A Centre exploring these same ideas called "New Economics" can be seen on their web site. **The way you understand these larger social factors and how you adapt and allow for them rests with you and the way you choose to live, "The Path to Wisdom lies Within"**

INDIVIDUAL CAUSES.

Lifestyle Diet and Eating Regime. The most important factor in establishing good health and freedom from disease is your own choice of lifestyle, diet and your way of cooking and eating: "Man ist was Man isst" a German adage meaning "one is what one eats"

Your diet and eating regime is probably the only thing about which you have complete choice.

Susceptibility to disease from one's inheritance. Inheritance is an important factor in determining our susceptibility to disease, it is an **individual** susceptibility: we are all different. This is especially true in considering non food substances including tobacco the effect of which varies considerably from individual to individual according to their susceptibility, which partly depends on inheritance. The theory of susceptibility has recently been proven by a team of Canadian researchers led by Dr. Skamen who showed that the tubercular terrain (a susceptibility to have tubercular diseases) is a reality when they identified the responsible gene on chromosome II. The tubercular terrain is just one of several inherited susceptibilities. (15)

Self Awareness. Your state of mind on a daily basis, the quality of your thought patterns and emotional responses is important to your overall health. "When some people talk about all the days of their life—they spell it with a 'z'."

Breath awareness is important as a part of healthy living. Many overweight people routinely breathe through their mouths, which detracts from optimum health. Deep breathing will ensure a thorough gas exchange giving the body optimum oxygen and expulsion of carbon dioxide. The whole body benefits by this, including the digestive system. Balanced

<u>Breathing</u> *by making the inbreath and the outbreath equal in length (each having the same count) assists the mind to be calm and relaxes the body.*

6

The Role of Medicine: Cure and prevention

"Many of the health gains achieved during the nineteenth and early twentieth centuries were the consequence not of advances in medical science, but of improvements in nutrition and sanitation" (6) The Sanitary Engineer is responsible for the cure of many infections, including Cholera and Typhoid rather than vaccinations as is claimed. Several of these diseases were in decline thanks to better living conditions before their vaccine was introduced

Medical trials and research has a flaw in its basic assumptions. This is the belief that we are all the same, that we are all identical like mice and other animals. For each species animals have a group spirit or pattern of expression, humans have an individual spirit which makes us uniquely different one from another. Our susceptibility to disease and to medical agents differs according to each individual, one thing suits some individuals but not others

Different individual susceptibility explains the inevitable conflicts around any trial of any medicine or treatment and the conflicting results from various trials and the subsequent argument and disagreement about them. A trial successful with some is often believed to give similar benefit for everyone, which is never the case.

"Hence whenever there is one trial that shows that drug A is better than drug B, there is nearly always another which show the exact opposite" (7)

The National Health Service

There is wide recognition that medical doctors practice modern advanced medicine with skill and integrity to the highest standard. The system is at fault not the doctors; it breaks down because of overreliance on the drug industry and **a bias among legislators and the public alike, to expect welfare from outside of one's own choices to ensure health and well being, this breeds a culture of reliance, dependence and impotence. No amount of external medical intervention of any kind can correct a failure to live and eat healthily. External agents of disease do indeed exist but individual susceptibility to them varies widely. This susceptibility depends on all the factors mentioned but the one thing we have control over is our choice of life style, diet and eating habits.**

Suppression. The whole concept of beneficial medical research based on modern science is compromised whenever treatments are suppressive ie. when they aim to cure symptom syndromes, which are end-products of disease and do not treat causes which are found in the context of the whole life style and life cycle of each individual. **Supression is not confined to any one approach to treatment whether conventional or alternative. Suppression is an intention, you may suppress detrimentally with homoeopathy, acupuncture etc as well as with conventional medical treatment. If you intend to remove the end product of illness rather than to treat the causes any method you use will be detrimental.**

A widely publicised message recently seen on posters around the country states that the following diseases have been cured; Diphtheria then Polio then Typhoid then Cholera then, rather laughably, T.B. In fact these diseases have been suppressed by treating the end symptoms and not their causes, this leads to more serious, more deeply seated diseases becoming fashionable, like cancer, heart diseases and an ever increasing incidence of mental and drug dependence illnesses. Today 25% of the UK population suffers from some kind of mental illness. A strong indication that cancer, in particular, is a disease caused by modern living and diet is shown by Goldsmith. (4) There is no clearer example of suppression than the creation of AIDS from the frequent suppression of infections with antibiotics. It is essential to initiate changes to use treatments to remove the causes that generated the diseases in the first place.

Diseases naturally adapt to changes in their environment including suppressive medicines. An untreatable strain of XDR TB has been diagnosed.

The W.H.O. estimates that this strain accounts for about 2% of the world's 9 million TB cases. (Guardian 21/3/08) According to the Health Protection Agency cases of similarly resistant strains of TB nearly doubled between 1998 and 2005.

There are now ever increasing claims that research, for example stem cell work will help to cure diseases like Parkinson's, Diabetes and Alzheimer's to mention only three. The danger of treatments arising from this research is that they will be used supresively. **Whilst the fundamental causes of all disease remain unchanged treatment will continue to create a new generation of even more debilitating, deeper diseases continuing the present attack on the dignity, quality and independence of human beings.**

The study of Science of Mind (11) shows that the possibility of having a disease lies in individual's thoughts, attitudes and feelings.

Until society is improved by reforms in social justice, equality and correct information and also individuals take responsibility for their own diet and life style as suggested in this book the Nation's Health remains at risk.

Mass Imunisation

That vaccination can also cause more disease was recognized in a small way when American A.B.C. reported that the U.S. Government concedes that there may be a link between vaccines and autism (www blacklisted news.com/view. 2008).

Studies published by the World Health Organization in 1982 of trials in India over seven and a half years including 270,000 children concluded that the BCG vaccine against tuberculosis is ineffective. Many countries have since ceased the obligatory use of BCG

A definitive book by Dr. Richard Halvorsen, a British GP. (6) is a formidable treatise on the whole range of issues about vaccination.

He questions the need for some vaccines, dating their introduction to when the disease in question was already in decline. He also states with measles that,

"research suggests that there is truth in the view that catching measles is good for children."

Some of his findings include:

"Infectious Diseases are rarely a major public health problem unless they are able to thrive in conditions of poverty, malnutrition and poor sanitation."

"Looking back the killer diseases of a century ago have all but disappeared. But in their place we have chronic diseases such as arthritis, diabetes, asthma and exzema for which medicine has no cure."

In the chapter on the developing world, entitled 'Death by Vaccination':-*"If it is true that mass immunisation was introduced in the West without the proper controls that apply to other medication, then this has always been the case for the developing world."*

The chapter on research into vaccines shows how the research results are edited for publication: *"There are a lot of people who are afraid to publish work that will displease the Department of Health and Big Pharma"*

Misinformation and exaggeration about the seriousness and dangers of most vaccinated diseases are widespread also the Health Authorities in every country and World Organisations repeat, without scrutiny or rigorous enquiry, information supporting the drug industry's claims.

The final conclusion on a particularly controversial vaccine:

"We live supposedly, in a free and open society. This makes it all the more strange why it has been impossible to have a rational discussion about the risks, and benefits of the MMR vaccine without personal attacks and accusations of putting children's lives at risk."

Recently (September 2009), a vaccine claiming to cure Cancer has been announced, the likelihood of such an application offers the certainty of even more serious diseases, probably of a mental and emotional nature.

Dr. D. Grandgeorge M.D. of the Faculty of Medicine in Marseilles, a paediatrician and classical homoeopath with over forty years experience writes:

"The population is pressurized into having too many vaccinations, these days it is not unusual for a child to receive nineteen inoculations by the age of four months. Such excesses need to stop, because the immune disorders they produce are creating a generation of asthmatics. Asthma with its impeded respiration and congested lungs, tends to be blamed on environmental pollution and exposure to cigarette smoke but it is usually triggered by these first inoculations. I believe early vaccinations to be pointless, since up to the age of nine months the baby is protected by antibodies received via the mother's placenta before birth (whilst the antibodies received in breast milk protect the digestive tract against gastro-enteritis).

The whooping cough vaccine carries many risks (such as encephalitis) and can cause asthma, so should be reserved for children who are already socializing. I believe two injections to be more than enough to protect the child for the first year of life, the only time that whooping cough poses any threat. As for the BCG, whilst its efficacy remains unproven, it is a well known trigger for asthma and allergies. Finally the Measles, Mumps and Rubella vaccine; firstly it seems totally unnatural to put three such unrelated viruses together in a single vaccine, secondly, the vaccine does not protect for as long as the disease itself. Thirdly the fragility of these vaccines means they are easily destroyed, by exposure to heat for example. In other words, we run the risk of creating epidemics of measles, mumps and rubella among the adult population, who are much less able to tolerate such diseases. What's more, the eradication by vaccines of childhood diseases most likely affects and changes the immune system. This is a problem that affects the whole of society and should therefore be debated much more thoroughly than it has been to date. In my opinion, all other vaccinations are superfluous—meningitis, for example, occurs rarely and is usually reserved for children living in large groups. As for hepatitis B, it is hardly ever seen in a child under fourteen, also the genetically-produced vaccine does not yet carry a reliable guarantee of safety and has been linked with numerous serious side effects such as multiple sclerosis, sight problems, various auto-immune diseases and diabetes." (14)

7

Alternative Medicine

Alternative is in some ways a misleading term. There is no alternative to good medical treatment. Dr. Hahnemann, the founder of Homoeopathy, clearly states the imperative need for modern surgical and clinical methods as appropriate.(16) This is the correct treatment of the **end product** of disease. The prevention or treatment of early and intermediate stages of disease comes within the scope of alternative medicines like homoeopathy.

What is truly alternative is:

1. The understanding of the **causes** of disease.

2. The best means of treatment of the **origins and causes of disease.**

Science makes predictions by logic from stated premises. These predictions may be observed to be true or false in fact. Homoeopathic treatment is not based on speculation. Homoeopathy is empirical not theoretical, the symptoms any medicine will cure are known from carefully conducted trials on healthy people called provings.

The founder of Homoeopathy states this clearly:

"The unprejudiced observer well aware of the futility of transcendental speculation, which can receive no confirmation from experience ... takes note of nothing in every individual disease, except the changes in the health of body and of the mind"

The physician; "must not construct so called systems, by interweaving empty speculations and hypotheses concerning the internal essential nature of the origin of disease."

" ... everything that is conjectural, all that is mere assertion or imaginary should be strictly excluded; everything should be the pure language of nature, carefully and honestly interrogated" Oranon paras. 143/144.

That some professed homoeopathic practitioners do not comply with these principles is discussed by George Vithoulkas. (17)

Individualization of Treatment

Alternative medicine has given good service to many people both in prescribing curative medicine and in reducing reliance on conventional drugs, some of which are prescribed for the effects of drugs previously given. This is not to give a blanket condemnation of all conventional treatments. Patients are individuals; much conventional medicine is beneficial to some patients notably those requiring hormone replacements like insulin.

Homoeopathy offers the benefit of individualizing treatments on all levels, thus treating the causes not only the end products. This gives the choice to patients to select effective natural programmes of healthcare which may sometimes combine orthodox with the alternative.

Treating individuals as if they were all the same leads to a failure to ensure good treatment.

Antibiotics may sometimes be the chosen treatment, especially in serious conditions when homoeopathic remedies cannot quickly be found, however overuse of antibiotics can weaken the immune system. The ill effects of frequent reliance on antibiotics can be removed by a homoeopathic remedy called Gaertner. After antibiotics C-difficile bacteria which are the most harmful of the gut flora, will increase whilst the beneficial flora will decline. Your digestive process will be less efficient leading to low energy and weakness, in addition you become more prone to infections including M R S A and C-difficile. Conventionally probiotics (acidophilus) is employed with some slight benefit if taken daily. Far more effective is Gaertner which corrects both of these harmful effects of the overuse of antibiotic. Afterwards homoeopathic constitutional prescribing will strengthen the immune system so antibiotics will unlikely to be required again.

The Animal Kingdom—Experiments on animals.

Humans have evolved through the animal kingdom; respect for the animal kingdom is a natural instinct in all healthy humans. Under a homoeopathic medical regime it would be unnecessary to perform experiments on animals for drug tests; homoeopathic medicines are proven on healthy human beings giving a complete knowledge of their curative properties making animal experiments unnecessary.

When the nation decides to put aside the unthinking acceptance of propaganda from vested interests, narrow specialists and commercial dominance it will be possible to build up a medical regime without reliance on the torture and degradation of the animal kingdom, this would have a wide appeal.

The Future.

That alternative medicine can be curative is certain. The three main curative alternatives are Herbalism, Homoeopathy and Acupuncture. However, their effectiveness is dependent on the individual practitioner's abilities and knowledge. At this time alternative medicine is largely ungoverned, it is not difficult for opponents to discover unsafe or unethical practices by inferior practitioners. (17)

Homoeopathic practitioners treat exactly the same patients and diseases as do conventional practitioners.

A study published in *Pulse* magazine for GP's, *Pulse. co.uk 17 Feb 2009, shows conclusively favourable outcomes for alternative treatments.*Patients receiving homeopathic treatment reported an average 54% improvement in their health and well being, often after long standing conventional treatment had failed. CAM Pilot study 2008.

"Homoeopathy is the ideal medicine to accompany us on our life's path. It is nature's way of providing man with everything he needs in order to be healthy, by helping him overcome each of the obstacles in his way." D. Grandgeorge.(15)

Doctor' require and should have a disciplined medical training similar to a medical degree that they enjoy today but with the principles of classical homoeopathy taught from the outset of the degree. (This is found today in some universities in India, for example Bombay) This would require a rethink of what a medical degree should encompass. In addition the cost of health care would be reduced as homoeopathic medicines cost next to nothing.

Antagonism to Homoeopathy. The majority of great homoeopaths throughout its two hundred year's history were medical doctors. Two aspects of homoeopathy, which have been misrepresented, have generated opposition; one is the potentisation of medicines which has been confused with mere dilution. The other is the law of similars,

Potentisation involves a kinetic process of energy exchange which fits comfortably into modern science similar to field force physics. By this means the unique pattern of each remedy is transferred from the original into alcohol and water from which we can make preparations to prescribe. (19)

The law of similars. A simple illustration of this is to give an acid treatment for an acid condition rather than giving an alkali treatment which is contrary.

These two things have led many doctors to begin a study of homoeopathy with a view to discredit it once and for all. These open minded people, once they learned the principles and practice of homoeopathy became dedicated practitioners and teachers.

All open minded enquiries into the efficacy of classical homoeopathic medicine have proved favourable. Attacks on homoeopathy by medical doctors comes from fear, their whole philosophy as well as their livelihoods appears to be threatened and undermined. Support in this antagonism from the commercial drug companies compounds its force.

Complementary Medicine.

Complementary describes various practices which are effective in relieving symptoms, of palliation and of modifying a disease process. These include reflexology, cranio-sacral osteopathy, yoga therapy, metamorphic technique tai chi and manipulative treatments like chiropractics and Bowen technique. All of these and others are beneficial if practiced with care and skill, they may improve your life style and level of health and with some patients are fully curative.

Deep seated, long established disease usually requires a more profound approach offered by homoeopathy which is especially able to cure disease having its origins in inheritance even more so than acupuncture or herbalism.

8

Eating your way to health

The choice of food and drink eaten as your staple diet, the quality as well as quantity, which are interconnected, is an important factor in determining you health. Equally important is the way you prepare and eat your food. Ready meals and convenience food is harmful, for example trans fats included in the manufacture of deep fried foods, margarine and baked goods like cakes and biscuits are a strong cause of heart disease which doctors are pressing to ban.(21)

Observing nature leads to the theory of YIN and YANG. At the Poles it is extremely cold which is Yin, the only foods nature provides are meat and fish which are both yang especially meat. Near the equator it is very hot which is yang, here nature provides rich juicy foods and oils which are yin. These observations of nature are the basis for Macrobiotics (great living), which describes old traditional family methods of food preparation and cooking uncontaminated by commercial interests or by the influence of theories far distanced from nature.

<u>Climate and Latitude</u> These have a vital role to play in choosing which foods and type of cuisine is healthy for you. It is inadvisable to eat much food from distant latitudes which is only suitable for those who live in that climate. In addition there is an adverse impact on the carbon footprint.

<u>Enhancing your Digestion</u> **Chew Well.** This is the first and most important aid to a healthy diet and body. (Gladstone used to advocate giving 32 chews for each mouthful) this chewing aids the whole of the digestive tract. Chewing your food until it is close to becoming liquid enhances digestion and satisfies the appetite. Food swallowed after only a little chewing does not satisfy appetite and burdens the next stages of digestion which as a result may be incomplete; this leads to the desire for more food than the body needs for nutrition and satisfaction.

Eat a little raw food before every cooked meal. (I frequently add young dandelion leaves or sorrel from the garden to my starter salad)

With all salads use lemon juice rather than vinegar in the dressing.

Do not drink during eating; this dilutes the digestive juices whilst chewing. Only good quality tea and coffee in moderation is advisable green tea is preferred. It is currently fashionable to drink much water, drinks are yin, the kidneys have to process all liquids and should not be burdened with much liquid. Only drink genuine natural mineral or spring water. Tap water has harmful additives like fluoride. Soft drinks contain sweeteners and additives.

Be Brown It is essential to use only unrefined food, white refined food encourages overeating. It does not contain the nutrients our body requires, you therefore still feels hungry after eating what should be enough. Whole food contains trace elements, minerals and roughage all of which are required by the body to function healthily. Many of these ingredients are taken out and then sold to the gullible in the form of supplements, for example iodine which is found in unrefined sea salt, often this is purchased as a supplement to assist the thyroid in overweight persons also commercial salt is emasculated and of little value, unrefined sea salt is preferred. In addition refined white food is more difficult to chew thoroughly; it dissolves more quickly and is swallowed too soon for good digestion. For both these reasons over reliance on refined food is a significant cause of obesity.

Sugar.

Natural sugars are found in fruit and vegetables. Refined sugar distorts the ability to taste natural sugars; brown sugar of any kind is not significantly different from white sugar. Refined sugar, above all other refined foodstuffs, has probably the most deleterious effect on our health compounding all the bad effects of white refined foods, yet sugar beet growing is subsidised by the Government so that we pay taxes to encourage something which is harmful. Gradually eliminating all refined sugar from your diet will give you an enhanced appreciation of the natural taste of whole, fresh food revealing a new pleasure in life as well as enhancing your health.

Whole Food.

There is no need to peel, and scrape vegetables, throw away very little. Wash and scrub vegetables. You will never have to buy another stock cube; stock can be made from the greens you may have rejected in the past. The water from cooked vegetables contains valuable minerals and makes excellent stock in cooking and baking.

The use of artificial fertilizers and growth hormones drives deep into the soil natural minerals and nutrients which our food needs. The farming industry is boastful about producing cheap food, unfortunately this encourages the purchase of more than is needed and this cheap food is inferior to real, organic food.

> "Industrialization of agriculture has sometimes increase yields, but it has also destroyed the very land we depend on.
>
> When we talk about cheap food it is worth remembering that more often than not, we have paid twice for it—through our taxes, via subsidies, and over the counter." (4)

There is pressure on merchandisers to sell this glut and many offer bigger or double portions for the same price, restaurants are more and more offering bigger portions. This leads to the phenomenon of massive waste which we now see in western countries. (A recent estimate is that £40 billions worth of food is wasted in Britain each year)

What is appropriate to each one of us is unique. For example someone who works physically hard in their occupation requires a different diet from one who sits at a desk each day, both in quantity and type of food, but not in quality and not different from the other important principles here given.

Organics. There are many misconceptions about organic foods, they are food actually, food comes from growing not from industry; Foodstuffs coming from the "farming industry" encourage poor health and overeating. Food which involves disrespect of its source is unhealthy, whether it is cruelty involved in rearing battery hens and other animals, or by the use of artificial fertilizers, or from farm fishing. How our vegetables and animal live is most important, as is how they die.

Taste. Organic foods taste so much better, it is sometimes argued that it tastes no different; initially this may be accurate but after a few days the taste buds adapt and the improved taste becomes palpable. Your taste requires a little time to adapt; this is more obvious when taken into account with my other eating and cooking recommendations.

<u>Cost</u>. Although the price of organic is a little more expensive at point of purchase compared with junk foods, this higher cost is a delusion. First, less is discarded in preparation. Second less is eaten as organic food is more satisfying and fulfilling, this in conjunction with chewing well. Third what proportion of your disposable income do you spend on food? Consider you rent/mortgage, holidays, transport, entertainment, alcohol etc. How important do you consider your health.

Purchasing non organic factory foods and those brought long distances by air and ship plus costs arising from merchandising and advertising add up to substantial social costs not reflected in the prices you pay. These costs are imposed upon you in other ways.

Balanced Meals. Meals should consist of the main component like game, fish, a small quantity of organic meat or a vegetable option like falafel, tempura (deep fried battered vegetable pieces) stuffed vine leaves and most important a whole grain or bread made from their flour, grains like short grain rice,(long grain is grown in warmer latitudes) buckwheat (particularly good for those who have much physical activity in their work or leisure) bulgar, oats, cous cous, such grains or breads should make up about a third of the meal, which ensures a balanced diet. Some unleavened bread is a good addition to your diet. Essentially moderate quantities should make up each meal. "quantity changes quality".

Key Ingredients. With every meal there are three key ingredients salt, oil and a good quality soya sauce, usually bought under the Japanese names of Shoyu or Tamari, this is used in cooking not added to you plate.

Salt. The body needs salt. Commercial salts are refined and harmful; some important elements are removed in their refinement. It is essential to use unrefined sea salt in cooking, do not add salt to your meal on the plate, gomasio may be added beneficially, this is a mix of sesame seeds and salt which has no harmful effects yet gives a suitable and tasteful seasoning. The salt is coated with sesame oil and is more easily digested and adds flavour. (24)

Oil. Use only cold pressed oil, when oil is extracted under heat more oil is obtained but the heat process destroys essential ingredients like proteins, minerals and trace elements.

Tahini. This is cream made from sesame seeds. It can replace butter in several uses and is also good to add a little on your plate to cooked grains and sautéed vegetables.

Pulses. of all kinds preferably organic and good quality are a valuable part of many meals, grains and pulses eaten together can release more protein.

Oat Cakes. Original oat cakes are an unleavened bread of great merit in any diet, Available in most shops are oatcake biscuits which make an excellent food to use instead of, or with sweet biscuits.

Miso This is soya fermented with either rice or barley. It provides protein. It has several uses in your cooking and diet, it should not be added whilst the dish is still cooking, add just after, so as to preserve valuable enzymes.

Seaweeds (sea vegetables). Most parts of the British coastline yield samphire, dulce and other sea foods. These have iodine and minerals and make a nutritious and tasty ingredient, They are readily found under Japanese names like nori, wakame and kombu.

Lemon Juice. This is an excellent cleanser which dissolves deposits in the joints, it is used in salad dressings and some drinks for example lemon barley water with honey which is a mainstay of any short term cleansing diet.

Things to be avoided:

VINIGAR, however fancy, wine, cider, or any other vinegar: this acid is too strong to be easily assimilated; for salad dressings use lemon juice and cold pressed oil together with seasoning to taste.

PICKLES and yeast products like marmite.

MOLLASES and other products from sugar: Organic honey in small amounts is a good substitute.

CREAM: Use natural, plain yoghurt instead.

Utensils and Cooking Pots. Aluminium utensils are harmful to your digestive system. A parliamentary enquiry after the war produced a minority report wishing to ban them after hearing the evidence. The availability of cheap aluminium at this time swayed the majority to recommend their acceptance. Enamel and iron are good; anaemia was a far less prevalent complaint when iron utensils were more commonly used. Teflon coated pans of any kind are best avoided also, grease-proof paper is preferable to cling film or aluminium foil. Glass and stainless steel are good to use. There is also available an unglazed pot with a lid in which potatoes are cooked in the oven with nothing added, this produces potatoes similar to those cooked as the Irish do on an open peat fire. A stainless steel pressure cooker is also a great asset in cooking. Use only wooden spatulas or spoons in cooking. In the orient it is considered harmful to put metal in the mouth so ceramic spoons and wooden chop sticks are favoured.

Cooking Methods.

Steaming is a good way to cook, less water is required than with boiling, but in either case the water should not be discarded, this is where minerals and other nutrients are stored.

Sauté (stir frying) Cut the vegetables into small pieces and place in the heated oil which seals in the nutrients and taste, add a little tamari, this gives the perfect balance of yin to yang. When vegetables are a part of any meal including soups or casseroles it is beneficial to first sauté them. Potatoes, aubergines and tomatoes are very watery, yin, and are best cooked separately and in moderation.

Deep Frying. Oil is yang this balances the yin vegetables.

Vegetarianism

Meat is very yang and too much meat eating leads to illness and aggressive attitudes. Fish has since ancient times been a preferred source of protein, especially with spiritual leaders and teachers. (8).

Vegetarian diets can be less than ideal. Sometimes the diet errs in eating too much dairy food, cooking over-rich sauces and using too many tomatoes and rich fruit and vegetables from distant climes. A vegetarian regime, when combined with the other advice given here can give you a healthy and active life. Always prefer wild rather than farmed fish and organic meat. Game also is a tasty and healthy meat option. Some spiritual teachers have observed that becoming a vegetarian is applicable only to a relatively few of the total population at present. The majority of mankind is working on (1) becoming individualized and (2) learning true thought in the brain. Meat is one of the means by which we are being aided in this evolutionary development.

I recall being told that Their Conference Centre was "low meat" I immediately envisaged roast snakes, barbecued lizard etc. It was not what they meant.

Food Additives and Behavioural Problems in Children

There is a growing recognition that food additives create in children behavioural problems like hyperactivity, aggression, attention deficit disorders and others. This has long been known to many parents who have found a remarkable improvement when additives and colourings ie: junk food was avoided. Alternative therapists and doctors have also seen many dramatic improvements from this change in diet. Recent research in which The Food Standards Agency was involved showed that certain artificial colourings and preservative confirmed this fact. (21) How much violence and aggression in adults would be reduced by a similar change? Some research conducted at Aylesbury prison did confirm that this connection was in fact true. (23) Self harm was also implicated in the findings.

"a growing body of research demonstrates the impact of diet on mental health, and there is also growing evidence to link diet to anti-social and criminal behaviour." (4)

THE CAUSES OF OBESITY

1. *Eating foods from all over the world as well as an enormous array of prepared foods means our liver does not have to synthesise new*

molecules but finds them in our diet without effort. The liver becomes lazy and we often become sluggish and fat.

2   The failure to chew well enough the food we eat.

3   Eating white refined breads, grains and pasta.

4   Using too many products like pickles and chutneys which contain sugar and vinegar, which over-stimulate the appetite.

5   Cheap food which means too much is eaten.

6   Drinking the wrong kind of drinks containing sugar or equally harmful sweeteners, and flavourings. Squeeze your own oranges.

Morgan Spurlock conducted an experiment where he ate only McDonald meals for a month. This demonstrated medically how his health seriously deteriorated. This is shown in the film "Super Size Me"

Overweight and Obesity.

Attempts are made to excuse bad eating regimes and choices by laying the blame outside of individual responsibility. The two main excuses are usually Metabolism and Hormones.

Metabolism

People are individually different and your metabolism is unique to you. The ductless glands secrete hormones which act as chemical messengers. One of these ductless glands is the thyroid gland which controls metabolism: under-function of the thyroid leads to a tendency to add weight easily; the opposite condition leads to a thinner body and underweight. **The secretion of hormones is balanced and encourages health when your mental and emotional activity is harmonious, peaceful and positive.** Cultivating these qualities and a good diet can prevent excesses one way or the other. The thyroid gland can also be affected favourably by homoeopathic and herbal medicines specific to the gland and its healthy functioning.

Hormones

Modern farming methods, employ hormones in arable, animal and fish farming. These hormones are long lived and come into the water supply and into waste products that go into soil, rivers and seas. These hormones are absorbed into the body from conventional food and diet. In recent years fertility abnormalities have been recorded in nature and there is an increase in infertility problems in people. (4 page 61) It may be that hormonal imbalance leading to a tendency to obesity can be limited and eventually corrected by eating a good diet free from hormones.

"The food industry uses roughly 400 million tonnes of chemicals in tens of thousands of varieties every year. Most have never been tested for their effects on health and environment." (4)

Dieting and Diets The reason for special diets is to achieve a specific purpose. When that purpose is accomplished the diet should be changed. Many people eat all the time a diet which should have been restricted to a limited period. Reference 25 gives recipes for safe, cleansing diets **including one for obese people**.

VITAMINS AND SUPPLEMENTS

Adding supplements to your body's economy is only necessary in advanced stages of deterioration from bad living, diet, and eating habits. In reasonable health the body will suppress its natural defensive processes if artificial supplements are regularly added. **This is part of nature's law of economy and adaptation.** This argument applies equally to the addition of fluoride in toothpaste and water supplies, fluoride has effects on human feelings and behaviour, a fact demonstrated by trials on healthy individuals during homoeopathic "provings" of Fluoride.(14) *The same considerations apply to vitamins. The first vitamin was made from the outer layers of rice discarded when polishing rice to make it white. Eating whole, brown, foods ensures that the body has all the minerals and trace elements which it uses to obtain all the needs vitamins have been found to provide.* **The exact same benefits claimed**

for vitamins and supplements are available from simple healthy eating habits, as advocated in this book.

Diet, vitamins and supplements in ill health. It has been found that in certain disease conditions the advice on diet, supplements and vitamins given here can be varied with benefit, for example in gout drinking more is beneficial, and in other diseases certain vitamins are beneficial.

9

Conclusion

It is unfair and unrealistic to put the whole burden of cure on the medical profession. Cure must be directed towards the causes of ill health. The State must re-align its policies and regulation to ensure individual responsibility for health and for the costs of treatment of illness brought on by self abuse, unhealthy diet and life style. Individuals must be made responsible for their own well being and state of health. Medical education and training must be widened to include alternatives and individualisation of treatment.

<u>Necessary Reforms</u> "We must redesign our welfare system so that it values and works with the vital operating systems, natural and social, and it will need a new perspective on the market economy" (10)

First of all It is necessary for government policies on tax and subsidies to farming and fish quotas to be changed away from erroneous views of what it is good and acceptable to eat to policies to promote health. The reforms that are needed are detailed in Goldsmith (4).Direct individual contribution to the cost of any medical treatment will have to be made under certain circumstances, first for those who are obviously suffering from self inflicted illness by eating badly and other regular habits of misuse or abuse of their body. It cannot be expected to implement this at once, it can only be implemented after a program of information, education and consultation so what is involved is universal

Inequality of income. The excesses of this phenomenon have to be modified by the reform of the tax system and the control of excessively high incomes.

POSTSCRIPT

The urgency and necessity of these changes is shown by recent proposals by the government: "our aim is to give people the help and advice they need to adopt a healthy life style" and "The Health Minister subscribes to the view that public health should be more a matter of personal responsibility than government action and too much emphasis has been put on treating illness in the NHS rather than preventing it in the first place" (Health Department Spokesman) Guardian 13,11.10

Five Networks are to be established which involve the food and drink industries, the alcohol business and also behaviourist advisers, this latter inspired by a book from The Chicago Business School. (23)

Doubts are cast on achieving results "Since the priority of the drinks industry, for example, is to make money for shareholders while public health demands a cut in consumption" Guardian 13.11.10. "In public health the track record of industry has not been good. Obesity is a systemic problem and industry is locked in to thinking of its own narrow interests" Professor Tim Lang Advisory Comity on Obesity.

Cleansings and Healthy diets.

No matter what we eat we are always on a diet. Our choice of diet, then, should be appropriate to our individual needs based on the nature of daily activity and the general state of mind and body.

As a person accumulates fat the organs of the body deposit waste material and toxins in the fatty tissue. The liver is the great manufacturing unit of the body. It takes from the bloodstream foodstuffs that have been eaten and reassembles them to make molecular structures needed by the body. This process was essential in earlier times when the range of our diet was limited and more suitable to our way of life.

When we regularly eat foods from all over the world as well as an enormous array of prepared foods our liver does not have to synthesise new molecules but finds them in our diet without effort. The liver becomes lazy and we often become sluggish and fat. A cleansing diet provides an opportunity for the liver to go to work again, as it should. The liver must draw on body accumulation of fat and synthesize molecules for its needs from fruit and vegetables in a cleansing diet.(25)

References In The Text

1. *Guardian 4 June 2010.*

2. *"The End of Overeating" David A. Kessler. Penguin 2009*

3. *Science Daily Jan 12 2009.*

4. *The Constant Economy by Zac Goldsmith*

5. *Mental Health, Resilience and Inequalities. The Mental Health Foundation.*

6. *The Truth about Vaccines by Dr. Richard Halvorsen. Penguin.*

7. *The Truth About Drug Companies by Marcia Angell. Random House*

8. *Felicity Lawrence. "Eat Your Heart Out"*

9. *The Spirit Level by richard Wilkinson and Kate Pickett. Penguin Books*

10. *Stiglitz Report The Commission on Measurement of Economic Performance and Social Progress. Launched in February 2008 by the French President.*

10 Mental Health Resilance and Inequalities The Mental Health Foundation.

11. A Review of the teachings of "Science of Mind" available from the author :www.ernestroberts.co.uk

12. D. Hamilton "How Your Mind Can Heal Your Body"

13. Richard Bentall "Doctoring the Mind Why Psychiatric Treatments Fail"

14. DidierGrandgeorgeMD. TheSpiritofHomoeopathic Medicines

15 Didier Grandgeorge MD. Homoeopathic Remedies for the Stages of Life.

16 The Organon of Medicine by Samuel Hahnemann

17. British media attacks on homeopathy: Are they justified? By George Vithoulkas. "Homoeopathy" Journal of The Faculty of Homoeopathy, London 2008.

18. "The Role of Medicine: Dream, Mirage or Nemesis" by Thomas McKeown 1979

20. George Vithoulkasis currently directing research at The University of Athens, Greece to prove how homoeopathic remedies work.

21. Report of Harvard Medical School published in The British Medical Journal March 2010.

22. McCann et al, The Lancet 2007; 370: 1560-1567.

23. Nudge: Improving Decisions About Health Wealth and Happiness. Richard Thaler and Cass Sunstein

24. The Art of Just Cooking by Lima Oshawa.

25. Cleansing Diet details on www.ernestroberts. co.uk

Other Recommended Sources.

A New Model of Health and Disease George Vithoulkas

Heal Thyself by Edward Bach Chapter 1.

The Creation of Health by Caraline Myss and C.N.Shealy.

Homoeopathy Principles and Practice by Ernest Roberts.

Not on the Label by Felicity Lawrence. Penguin

A History of Money Medicine and Politics by Paul Goddard.

Medicines Patients and the Law by Margaret Brazier Penguin.

The Great Food Gamble by John Humphrys

The Prostate Care Cookbook Margaret Rayman et al.

Zen Macrobiotics and The Book of Judgement by George Ohsawa

Fast Food Nation. By Eric Schlosser. Penguin 2002

The End of Overeating. By David A. Kessler. Penguin 2008.

Gesch et.al. British Journal of Psychiatry, vol181 2002 pp.22-8.

The Web Sites: wisebrain.org. sciencedaily.com and neweconomics.org/programmes/well-being.

The Film "Super Size Me" by Morgan Spurlock

The Film "Fast Food Nation" Hanway and B B C Films.

www.ingramcontent.com/pod-product-compliance
Lightning Source LLC
Chambersburg PA
CBHW020403290526
45785CB00005B/2422